DRY MOUTH

The Signs and Causes of Dry Mouth: Going Beyond Just Thirst

CARL JUAN

Table of Contents

Introductory

Xerostomia, or "dry mouth," occurs when saliva production in the mouth is inadequate or absent altogether.

• Saliva lubricates the mouth and helps with things like speaking, chewing, and swallowing by keeping the mouth wet.

• Saliva provides enzymes that start the digestion process by breaking down food.

• Hygiene of the mouth and teeth: saliva washes away leftover food and microorganisms. It also prevents tooth decay by neutralizing acids and reducing sensitivity.

• Clear speaking depends on having enough saliva.

Many things might cause your mouth to dry out, from prescription drugs to health problems to poor eating habits to simply getting older. Dehydration, anxiety, radiation therapy, autoimmune illnesses, and the natural aging process are common causes of dry mouth, as are several drugs (such as antihistamines, antidepressants, and diuretics).

A dry or sticky mouth, increased thirst, trouble swallowing and talking, a sore throat, a hoarse voice, foul breath, and an increased risk of dental issues including cavities and gum disease are all possible symptoms of dry mouth.

Adjusting medications or treating underlying medical issues are common approaches to managing dry mouth. In the meanwhile, those who suffer from dry mouth can take measures to improve their symptoms by, for example, increasing their water intake, chewing sugar-free lozenges or gum, and practicing regular, thorough dental hygiene. Dentists may also prescribe saliva replacement therapy or suggest alternative therapies for patients with this issue.

CHAPTER ONE
Dry Mouth: Its Origins and Repercussions

Xerostomia, or dry mouth, is a condition that has a wide variety of potential causes and symptoms. Dry mouth can have a number of different causes and symptoms.

Dry Mouth's Root Causes:

• Dry mouth is a common adverse effect of many drugs, both prescription and over-the-counter. These may include antihistamines, decongestants, antidepressants, diuretics, and drugs for high blood pressure.

• Dry mouth can be a symptom of a number of different medical disorders. Some examples are diabetes, autoimmunity (as in Sjögren's syndrome), HIV/AIDS, dementia, and tremors (as in Parkinson's disease).

• Dry mouth can be a transient symptom of dehydration, which can occur from not drinking enough fluids or from illnesses that induce excessive fluid loss, like fever, sweating, vomiting, and diarrhea.

• Injury or damage to the nerves in the head and neck might have an effect on the salivary glands, causing them to produce less saliva.

- Radiation therapy for head and neck cancer can cause dry mouth by damaging the salivary glands.

- Dry mouth and other problems with oral health can be caused by tobacco usage.

- Saliva production might decrease with age for a variety of reasons.

- Dry mouth is a symptom of stress and anxiety, which can cause the body to produce less saliva.

Dry mouth symptoms include:

- the most noticeable symptom of dry mouth is the sensation that one's mouth is always dry or parched. This is annoying and may make it hard to eat, swallow, or even talk.

• An increase in thirst is a common symptom of dry mouth as the body attempts to replenish lost saliva.

• A sore or scratchy throat is a common symptom of dry mouth because swallowing causes discomfort.

4. A lack of saliva can dry out the vocal cords and cause a raspy voice.

• Because saliva helps cleanse the mouth and remove odor-causing bacteria, a lack of saliva can lead to bad breath (halitosis).

• Alterations in TasteSome people who suffer from dry mouth report that their sense of taste shifts, and they report tasting something metallic or harsh.

• Trouble Speaking and Swallowing: Dry mouth can make it hard to form words clearly and can cause you to have trouble swallowing liquids and food.

• Cavities, gum disease, and mouth sores are all made more likely in people with dry mouth because saliva isn't able to adequately coat and protect the teeth.

Dry mouth can have serious consequences for both oral and general health, so it's crucial to determine what's causing it and treat it. If you have persistent dry mouth, it's best to see a doctor or dentist to figure out what's causing it and what may be done about it. In the meanwhile, you can ease your symptoms by taking care of your mouth, drinking plenty of water, and chewing sugar-free lozenges or gum.

Dental Health Consequences

The condition known as xerostomia, or dry mouth, can have serious consequences for teeth and gums. The mouth, teeth, and gums rely heavily on saliva to stay in good condition. Several problems with dental health can result from dry mouth, which occurs when saliva production is inadequate or absent.

1. Saliva helps prevent tooth decay (cavities) by rinsing away debris, neutralizing acids, and delivering minerals like calcium and phosphate. Tooth decay is more likely to occur when there is insufficient saliva to protect teeth. Cavities are more common in those with dry mouth.

2. By controlling the population of bacteria in the mouth, saliva plays an important role in preventing gum disease. Gum diseases including gingivitis and periodontitis are more likely to develop when saliva production decreases.

3. Sores in the Mouth: A lack of lubrication in the mouth can cause irritation and the painful sores that many people know all too well.

4. Halitosis, or chronic bad breath, can be treated by increasing saliva production. Insufficiency in saliva production might lead to chronic foul breath.

5. A person's ability to eat healthily may be impacted by dry mouth since it makes it more difficult to chew and swallow food.

6. Reduced saliva production might cause a person to have unpleasant aftertastes or a dulling of their sense of taste.

7. Infections of the Mouth and Throat Oral thrush (candidiasis) is a fungal infection that can spread more easily if your mouth is dry.

8. **Denture** **Discomfort:** Individuals who wear dentures may feel increased discomfort and problems with denture retention when they have dry mouth.

9. Problems Pronouncing: Dry mouth, because it reduces saliva production, might cause problems pronouncing words.

10. Increased teeth sensitivity from dry mouth makes it unpleasant to consume hot or cold liquids and foods.

To lessen the impact of dry mouth on dental health, it is vital to address the underlying cause when possible. Medication changes, medical care, and identifying and modifying risk factors in one's lifestyle are all potential avenues for alleviating dry mouth. Individuals with dry mouth can take measures to ease symptoms and protect oral health, in addition to addressing the underlying cause.

• Drink a lot of water during the day to keep yourself from being dehydrated.

The use of sugar-free gum, lozenges, or saliva substitutes is recommended.

Brush and floss your teeth twice a day to keep your mouth healthy.

To assist prevent tooth decay, you should use fluoride toothpaste and mouthwash.

Dry mouth can be made worse by tobacco and alcohol use, so stay away from both.

• See a dentist regularly for expert dental treatment and guidance on coping with dry mouth.

For a thorough assessment and individualized advice to treat dry mouth and its effects on dental health, it is vital to consult a healthcare professional or dentist.

CHAPTER TWO
Health Issues and Treatments

Medical illnesses and drugs can both cause or exacerbate dry mouth, also known as xerostomia. Some common diseases and drugs that cause dry mouth are listed below.

Disorders and Illnesses

• Dry mouth and eyes are hallmarks of Sjögren's disease, an autoimmune condition that predominantly targets the glands responsible for producing saliva and tears.

• Dry mouth is a common complication of uncontrolled diabetes because high blood sugar levels reduce saliva production.

• Dry mouth is one of the many oral issues that can arise from having the human immunodeficiency virus (HIV) or acquired immunodeficiency syndrome (AIDS).

• Alzheimer's Disease: People with Alzheimer's disease may have dry mouth as a result of diminished saliva production.

- Dry mouth can be a side effect of Parkinson's disease and some of the drugs used to treat it.

- Dry mouth can be a side effect of several drugs used to treat hypertension (high blood pressure), including diuretics and beta-blockers.

- Dry mouth is a common side effect of antidepressants and other medications used to treat depression and anxiety.

- Damage to the salivary glands, especially after radiation therapy to the head and neck for cancer treatment, can lead to persistent dry mouth.

• Dry mouth has been linked to autoimmune diseases such as systemic lupus erythematosus (SLE) and rheumatoid arthritis.

• Dry mouth can be caused by cystic fibrosis, a genetic condition that can impact several bodily functions.

Medications:

• Antihistamines are a class of drugs commonly found in cold treatments and allergy medications like diphenhydramine (Benadryl).

• Saliva production can be inhibited by decongestants, a class of drugs often used in cold and allergy remedies.

• Dry mouth can be a side effect of some antidepressants, including tricyclics and selective serotonin reuptake inhibitors (SSRIs).

• Dry mouth is a common side effect of diuretics, which are commonly used to treat illnesses like high blood pressure and edema.

• Dry mouth is a common side effect of some antipsychotic medications.

- Dry mouth is a common side effect of opiate pain medications like morphine.

- Medications for high blood pressure: beta-blockers and other blood pressure medications can cause dry mouth.

- Medications used to prevent or treat nausea and vomiting may cause dry mouth in some people.

- Some antibiotics, including atropine, might have the unintended effect of drying out your mouth.

- Dry mouth can be a side effect of stimulants, such as the

amphetamines used to treat attention deficit hyperactivity disorder (ADHD).

Salivary gland function can be affected differently by various drugs and health situations. If you experience recurrent dry mouth, it's crucial to discuss it with your healthcare practitioner or dentist. To alleviate symptoms, they may suggest modifying medications or utilizing saliva replacements, but they can also help determine the underlying problem.

The symptoms of dry mouth, also known as xerostomia, can be managed and even improved upon by a number of different means. Both the underlying reasons (if at all feasible) and the discomfort of dry mouth must be treated. **Some strategies for relieving dry mouth:**

• Keep your mouth moist by drinking water regularly throughout the day. Consume water frequently, particularly before, during, and after eating.

• Chewing sugar-free gum or sucking on sugar-free lozenges can temporarily alleviate dry mouth by stimulating saliva production.

• Artificial saliva products, often known as saliva substitutes, are available without a prescription and can be used to keep the mouth moist. You may get these in sprays, gels, and rinses, among other formats.

• **Oral Hydration Gel:** Some people find oral hydration gels, which are specifically developed to alleviate dry mouth, beneficial in retaining moisture in the mouth.

• Use a humidifier in your bedroom, particularly at night, to avoid overnight dry mouth by adding moisture to the air.

• Dry mouth can be caused by consuming too much caffeine or alcohol, so cutting back on these substances is recommended.

• **Avoid Tobacco:** Smoking and using tobacco products can exacerbate dry mouth and have a negative impact on oral health. If you smoke, quitting can help your symptoms.

• If you suffer from dry mouth, try to limit your intake of spicy and salty foods. You could feel better if you cut back on these kinds of foods.

• Brush your teeth at least twice a day with fluoride toothpaste and floss once a day to keep your mouth healthy. If you want to avoid cavities and keep your teeth healthy, you should use a mouthwash without alcohol.

• You should see your dentist regularly for checkups and cleanings. Your dentist can check on the state of your teeth and gums, offer guidance on how to alleviate dry mouth, and suggest fluoride treatments or dental products specifically formulated to do so.

• Discuss with your doctor whether or not you think your medication could be causing your dry mouth. They might be able to modify your medication or suggest alternatives that cause less dry mouth.

• Some methods and physical activities may stimulate the salivary glands. If you need help implementing these strategies, talk to your doctor or dentist.

• Changes to the diet: eat more fruits and vegetables, which contain a lot of water, and other foods high in moisture. These may be useful in replenishing the moisture in your mouth.

- Prescription medications Your doctor may recommend prescription medications to stimulate saliva production if the condition is severe and non-prescription options have failed.

- Work with your doctor to effectively manage or treat any underlying conditions that may be contributing to your dry mouth.

It's essential to consult with a healthcare provider or dentist to identify the cause of your dry mouth and receive personalized recommendations for managing it. Comfort and oral health can be enhanced by treating both the symptoms and the underlying causes.

If your dry mouth (xerostomia) is severe or long-lasting and you haven't found relief from self-care or OTC remedies, it's time to see a doctor. There are a variety of professional treatments available for dry mouth, and your doctor or dentist may recommend one of them depending on the underlying cause and severity of your condition.

- If your doctor suspects that dry mouth is a side effect of a medication you're taking, he or she may suggest lowering the dosage or switching to one that is less likely to have this effect.

- Prescription Medications: Your doctor may recommend a course of treatment that includes the use of prescription medications to increase saliva flow. Pilocarpine (Salagen) and cevimeline (Evoxac) are two examples of such drugs. Some people who suffer from dry mouth may benefit from taking one of these medications, which are designed to increase saliva production.

• Artificial Saliva Products: Your dentist or healthcare provider may recommend prescription artificial saliva products that can provide more effective relief for dry mouth symptoms compared to over-the-counter options.

• Stimulating the salivary glands may be suggested in some situations to increase saliva flow. Methods of stimulation could range from electrical to mechanical.

• Oral Moisturizing Gels and Sprays: Your healthcare provider or dentist can provide guidance on specific oral moisturizing gels and sprays that can effectively alleviate dry mouth symptoms.

• Your dentist may advise you to get regular fluoride treatments or use a special fluoride toothpaste to protect your teeth from problems like cavities.

• Dry mouth can be managed with the help of oral appliances, which dentists can create specifically for their patients. Water or medication reservoirs that slowly release moisture into the mouth may be included in such devices.

• If your dry mouth was caused by radiation therapy for head and neck cancer, your doctors may recommend shielding the salivary glands during future sessions of radiation therapy.

• Biofeedback and counseling are two examples of behavioral techniques that can teach people how to better handle the stress and anxiety that can lead to dry mouth.

• Surgical procedures may be considered to treat severe cases of dry mouth caused by issues like blocked salivary ducts or damaged salivary glands. Possible solutions include reconstructing the salivary gland duct or removing the obstruction.

• Management or treatment of the primary medical condition may be necessary if dry mouth is a symptom of another disease or disorder, such as Sjögren's syndrome or diabetes.

It is crucial to coordinate your care with your doctor and dentist to determine the best course of professional treatment for you. With their help, you can determine the root of your dry mouth problem and get on the road to better oral health and a better quality of life.

CHAPTER THREE
Dry Mouth and Dietary Considerations

Nutritional considerations are essential for individuals with dry mouth (xerostomia) because a dry oral environment can increase the risk of dental problems and affect overall nutrition and well-being. Here are some dietary recommendations and things to think about if you suffer from dry mouth:

• The single most important thing you can do for dry mouth nutritionally is to drink plenty of water. Keep your mouth moist and aid digestion by drinking water frequently throughout the day. Sip water frequently, especially during meals.

• Both caffeine and alcohol can exacerbate dry mouth, so cutting back on these substances is recommended. Select non-alcoholic and caffeine-free drinks.

• Easier to chew and swallow are moist, soft foods, so opt for those. It may be easier to eat foods like soups, stews, yogurt, and those with sauces or gravies. Dry, crunchy, or salty foods can irritate your mouth and make your mouth feel even drier.

• Watermelon, cucumbers, and citrus fruits are just a few examples of the many water-rich fruits and vegetables you should eat. These may be useful for rehydrating your mouth.

• Gum and hard candy without added sugar can help relieve dry mouth by stimulating saliva production. In an effort to lessen the likelihood of tooth decay, you should seek out xylitol-sweetened products.

• When it comes to your teeth, it's best to steer clear of acidic and sugary foods and drinks. You should cut back on acidic foods and drinks like soda, fruit juice, and citrus. You should gargle with water after eating them.

• Lean meats, poultry, fish, tofu, and legumes are all great sources of protein that you should add to your diet. Tissue repair and general wellbeing can both benefit from protein.

• Dairy products, such as milk, yogurt, and cheese, are a good source of protein and calcium, and they can also reduce the acidity of the mouth.

• Some people who suffer from dry mouth find that using moistening agents or oral lubricants developed for this purpose alleviates their discomfort. These aids can reduce the difficulty of eating and swallowing.

• If dry mouth is limiting your diet, talk to your doctor about taking a multivitamin or other nutritional supplement. Essential nutrients may be harder to come by, but supplements can help. Consult your doctor to find out what supplements are safe for you to take.

• Whole grains, fruits, and vegetables are great examples of high-fiber foods that are beneficial to digestive health. If you have trouble swallowing, getting enough fiber in your diet may be especially important.

• Foods that are too hot, too spicy, or too salty should be avoided because they can irritate the mouth and make dry mouth symptoms worse. Eat less of them or stay away from them entirely.

• Maintaining regular mealtimes has been shown to improve saliva regulation. Maintaining a regular eating schedule may help your body better recognize and respond to hunger cues.

In order to get nutritional advice tailored to your needs and medical condition, it's best to work with a healthcare provider or registered dietitian. They can assist you in developing a diet that will alleviate your dry mouth while still providing you with the nutrients you need to maintain good health.

Conclusion

dry mouth, or xerostomia, is a condition characterized by reduced or insufficient saliva production in the mouth. Medications, health problems, dietary decisions, and natural aging are all potential causes. Tooth decay, gum disease, bad breath, and difficulties speaking and swallowing are just some of the oral health problems that can arise from having a dry mouth.

• Staying hydrated, using sugar-free lozenges or gum, and practicing good oral hygiene are all effective ways to combat dry mouth. An oral health care provider may suggest a medication change, prescription medications, or artificial saliva products for severe or persistent cases of dry mouth.

• Staying hydrated, selecting moist and soft foods, limiting caffeine and alcohol, and incorporating fruits, vegetables, and protein-rich foods into the diet are all helpful for people who suffer from dry mouth. Maintaining optimal health and preventing dry mouth requires concerted effort from patients, dentists, and medical professionals.

An individual's quality of life, oral health, and comfort level can all benefit from learning more about the causes, symptoms, and treatment options available for dry mouth.

THE END

9 798876 916754